SIMPLIFIED GUIDE ON

INTEGRATIVE MEDICINE AND MIND- BODY HEALING

Unlocking Wellness Through Holistic Approaches, Integrative Therapies, And The Power Of Mind- Body Connection

DR. ARIYA REYNA

CONTENTS

Copyright © 2023, By Dr. Ariya Reyna

All Rights Reserved

This book is protected by copyright law, and any unauthorized reproduction, distribution, or transmission of the contents, in whole or in part, without the prior written consent of the author and the publisher is prohibited.

DISCLIAMER

This book is intended for informational purposes only and is not a substitute for professional medical advice, diagnosis, or treatment. The information provided in this book is based on the author's research and personal experiences and is not meant to replace the advice of healthcare professionals.

Readers are encouraged to consult with their healthcare providers before beginning any new exercise, wellness, or health program.

The author and publisher of this book are not responsible for any specific health or allergy needs that may require medical supervision and are not liable for any damages or negative consequences from any treatment, action, application, or preparation, to any person reading or following the information in this book.

The content of this book is not intended to be a substitute for professional medical advice, diagnosis, or treatment. Always seek the advice of your physician or other qualified health provider with any questions you may have regarding a medical condition.

The author and publisher disclaim responsibility for any adverse effects that may result from the use or application of the information contained in this book.

References to specific products, services, or organizations do not imply endorsement or recommendation by the author or the publisher.

The inclusion of such references is for illustrative purposes only. Thank you for reading and respecting the terms outlined in this disclaimer.

CHAPTER ONE

Integrative Medicine Overview

Integrative medicine is a comprehensive approach to healthcare that integrates standard Western medicine with complementary and alternative therapies. It focuses on treating the full person — mind, body, and spirit — rather than simply symptoms. The objective is to attain maximum health and wellness by taking into account the specific circumstances of each individual and utilizing various therapy techniques.

In contrast to the traditional style of healthcare, which frequently focuses primarily on symptom relief through drugs or surgery, integrative medicine takes a wider approach. It acknowledges the interdependence of numerous areas of a person's life, including physical health, emotional well-being, lifestyle, and environment.

Personalized treatment is a core component of integrative medicine. Practitioners collaborate closely with patients to create customized treatment regimens that may involve a combination of traditional medicine, diet, mind-body practices, herbal medicines, and other complementary therapies. This patient-centered approach seeks to encourage individuals to actively participate in their health and well-being.

Perspectives On Integrative Approaches Throughout History

Integrative medicine has its origins in ancient healing practices from countries all over the world. Many ancient medical systems, like Ayurveda in India and traditional Chinese medicine (TCM), have long emphasized the need for internal balance and harmony as a basis for good health.

Integrative medicine gained popularity in the Western world in the late twentieth century. Dissatisfaction with mainstream medicine's limits, along with a growing interest in alternative medicines, resulted in a more inclusive approach to healthcare. Influential personalities such as Dr.

Andrew Weil were instrumental in popularizing integrative medicine in the United States.

Over time, research has proven the efficacy of various complementary medicines, further adding to integrative methods' popularity. Many medical institutions and healthcare professionals now provide integrative medicine services, recognizing the need to integrate the best of traditional and alternative methods.

Mind-Body Healing Principles

Integrative medicine emphasizes the interdependence of mental and physical health via mind-body healing. This method acknowledges that emotional and psychological elements can have a substantial influence on physical well-being and vice versa. Within the context of integrative medicine, many essential ideas guide mind-body healing:

1. The Mind-Body Connection: This notion recognizes the complex link that exists between mental and physical wellness. Physical problems can

be exacerbated or exacerbated by stress, worry, and negative thinking patterns, whereas good emotions and a calm mental state can encourage recovery.

2. Stress Reduction Techniques: Stress reduction techniques such as meditation, deep breathing, and mindfulness are frequently used in mind-body healing. These techniques not only aid with stress management but also contribute to general well-being by encouraging relaxation and mental clarity.

3. Support for Emotions and Spirituality: Integrative medicine recognizes the need to address the emotional and spiritual components of health. Providing emotional support, cultivating a sense of purpose, and supporting spiritual well-being may all contribute to a more comprehensive approach to rehabilitation.

4. Mindful Movement: Yoga and tai chi stress the connection of movement and breath, which promotes physical health while also improving mental concentration and emotional balance.

Health And Wellness On A Holistic Level

A basic concept in integrative medicine, holistic health, and wellness goes beyond the absence of disease and focuses on obtaining optimal well-being in all aspects of life. This approach understands that nutrition, exercise, mental and emotional states, social relationships, and environmental variables all have an impact on health.

1. Diet & Nutrition: Holistic health emphasizes the necessity of a nutritious and well-balanced diet. Food is seen not only as a source of energy for the body but also as a source of healing and vitality. Nutrition is critical in promoting the body's natural healing processes and avoiding sickness.

2. Physical Activity: Regular exercise is essential for overall health. It not only promotes physical fitness but also promotes mental and emotional well-being. Integrative medicine promotes a wide range of physical activities that are adapted to individual tastes and health requirements.

3. Mental and Emotional Well-Being: Holistic health acknowledges the influence of mental and emotional states on total wellness. To achieve emotional balance, practices such as meditation, psychotherapy, and stress management techniques are incorporated into holistic health treatments.

4. Strong social relationships and a supportive community are essential for holistic wellness. Positive relationships and a sense of belonging help with emotional well-being and even improve physical health.

5. Environmental Factors: Holistic health emphasizes the environment's impact on well-being. This covers air and water quality, exposure to chemicals, and the general influence of the environment on health.

Nutritional Role In Integrative Medicine

Nutrition is a cornerstone of integrative medicine, playing a critical role in health promotion and disease prevention. This nutritional approach goes beyond merely counting calories and takes into account food quality, individual dietary demands, and the possible therapeutic benefits of certain nutrients.

1. Entire Foods and Nutrient Density: Integrative medicine advocates eating entire, minimally processed foods that are high in nutrients. Choosing nutrient-dense meals gives the body with the vitamins, minerals, and antioxidants it needs to function properly.

2. Tailored nutrition programs: Integrative medicine practitioners create tailored nutrition programs because they recognize that each person has different nutritional needs. These plans consider characteristics such as age, gender, health status, and any pre-existing medical issues.

3. Integrative medicine involves the notion of functional foods, which are foods that provide health advantages in addition to basic nourishment. Berries with antioxidant qualities, fatty fish high in omega-3

fatty acids, and anti-inflammatory medicines are some examples.

4. Nutritional Supplements: Nutritional supplements may be advised in some circumstances to treat particular deficiencies or to maintain general health. Vitamins, minerals, and herbal supplements customized to an individual's needs might be included.

5. Integrative medicine understands the relevance of gut health in overall health. Better digestion, immunological function, and even mental health have all been linked to healthy gut flora. Probiotics and a fiber-rich diet help to maintain a healthy gut ecology.

CHAPTER TWO

Botanical Therapies And Herbal Medicine

Herbal medicine, an important component of integrative medicine, uses plants and plant-derived chemicals to enhance health and prevent or treat sickness. This method has profound historical origins and is found in many traditional healing systems across the world.

1. Herbal treatments: Integrative medicine includes a variety of herbal treatments for a variety of health issues. Plants with immune-boosting, anti-inflammatory, and soothing effects, such as echinacea, ginger, and chamomile, are often utilized.

2. Individualized Herbal Protocols: Herbal therapies, like other areas of integrative medicine, are frequently tailored to the individual. Factors such as the person's constitution, health state, and potential prescription interactions are considered.

3. Nutraceuticals: Nutraceuticals are nutritional supplements produced from plants that are commonly used in integrative medicine. Extracts from turmeric, green tea, and ginkgo biloba, for example, are renowned for their potential health advantages.

4. Traditional Wisdom and Scientific Research: When proposing herbal remedies, integrative medicine practitioners frequently draw on both traditional wisdom and scientific research. While traditional plant applications give significant insights, scientific research helps us understand the efficacy and safety of herbal treatments.

5. While herbal therapy is usually regarded as safe, integrative medicine practitioners are aware of potential interactions with medicines as well as individual sensitivities. Individuals must notify their healthcare professionals about any herbal supplements they are taking for their care to be thorough and safe.

Traditional Chinese Medicine And Acupuncture

Acupuncture is a therapeutic practice used in Traditional Chinese Medicine (TCM) that includes putting small needles into certain sites on the body to improve balance and restore the flow of energy, known as Qi. TCM, which has thousands of years of history, provides a unique viewpoint on health and illness.

1. TCM principles: TCM sees the body as a complex system of linked channels through which Qi, or life energy, flows. Acupuncture is used to restore harmony and balance to the flow of Qi, which is thought to contribute to sickness.

2. Acupuncture points are precise areas on the body where needles are put to alter the flow of Qi. These points are said to connect to energy lines or meridians, and activating them can have a variety of medicinal benefits.

3. Acupuncture is used to treat a wide range of health ailments, including pain management, stress reduction, digestive problems, and reproductive health. Its holistic approach is consistent with integrative medicine ideas, addressing not just symptoms but also the underlying imbalances that contribute to illness.

4. Individualized Treatment Plans: Acupuncture treatment plans, like those of other integrative medicine modalities, are frequently customized. To personalize acupuncture treatments to the patient's exact needs, practitioners assess the patient's general health, specific symptoms, and any underlying imbalances.

5. While the foundations of TCM diverge from Western biological conceptions, there is significant scientific interest and study in acupuncture. Acupuncture may alter a variety of physiological processes, including neurotransmitter release and immune system regulation, according to research.

Finally, integrative medicine is a complete, patient-centered approach to treatment. This concept seeks to address the complexities of human health and wellness by embracing ideas of mind-body healing, holistic health, nutrition, herbal medicine, and acupuncture. As research supports the usefulness of integrative techniques, they are expected to play a larger role in influencing the future of healthcare.

Ayurveda: Ancient Wisdom In Contemporary Medicine

Ayurveda, an ancient medical system that originated in India over 5,000 years ago, is gaining popularity in modern medicine as a holistic approach to treatment. The term "Ayurveda" comes from Sanskrit and means "knowledge of life," stressing the interdependence of the body, mind, and spirit. Unlike Western medicine, which frequently focuses on treating symptoms, Ayurveda aims to address the underlying causes of illness and promote general well-being.

The belief in three doshas - Vata, Pitta, and Kapha - at the heart of Ayurveda represents diverse combinations of the five elements (earth, water, fire, air, and ether) found in all living things. Each person is said to have a distinct constitution, or Prakriti, that impacts their physical, mental, and emotional qualities. Ayurvedic practitioners customize remedies to balance these doshas, restore harmony, and prevent sickness.

Ayurveda takes a holistic approach to treatment, including dietary recommendations, herbal therapies, yoga, meditation, and cleansing techniques. Ayurvedic medicine considers nutrition to be an important part, with specific suggestions based on one's constitution and present state of imbalance. Ayurvedic therapies frequently include herbal formulations, such as turmeric for its anti-inflammatory effects or ashwagandha for stress reduction.

Ayurveda is progressively being incorporated into complementary and alternative medical techniques in modern healthcare. Its emphasis on tailored treatment strategies and illness prevention corresponds to a growing interest in holistic health. Because of Ayurveda's popularity, Ayurvedic practitioners and conventional healthcare specialists have joined forces to provide patients with a more complete approach to their health.

Healing Touch And Energy Medicine

Energy medicine refers to a variety of therapies that focus on the body's energy systems to facilitate healing. The concept that interruptions or imbalances in the body's energy flow lead to physical, mental, and emotional disorders is at the heart of these practices. Healing Touch, a therapeutic strategy in which the practitioner uses their hands to detect and balance the patient's energy field, is a key part of energy medicine.

Healing Touch is based on ancient healing traditions and the belief that the body has an innate power to heal itself. Gentle, non-invasive procedures are used by practitioners to impact the body's energy field, which is supposed to extend beyond the physical body. Healing Touch attempts to enhance the body's natural healing processes by fostering balance and harmony in the energy field.

Energy medicine research is underway, to determine its potential advantages for various health issues. While some opponents contend that the mechanics underlying energy medicine are unclear, proponents point to its good influence on stress reduction, pain management, and overall well-being. Healing Touch is frequently used alongside traditional therapies in integrative healthcare settings, recognizing the potential synergies between energy medicine and orthodox medical techniques.

CHAPTER THREE

Meditation And Mindfulness Practices

Mindfulness and meditation are widely recognized as effective strategies for increasing mental health and well-being. These practices, which have their roots in ancient contemplative traditions, include fostering awareness, attention, and presence in the present moment. Mindfulness and meditation are recognized as important components of holistic healthcare in integrative medicine, with the potential to improve physical, emotional, and mental health.

Mindfulness, which derives from Buddhist traditions, entails paying conscious attention to the present moment without judgment. This practice is frequently included in several therapeutic modalities, such as mindfulness-based stress reduction (MBSR) and mindfulness-based cognitive therapy (MBCT), which have demonstrated benefits in the treatment of diseases such as anxiety, depression, and chronic pain.

Meditation, a wide phrase that encompasses many contemplative activities, seeks to produce a state of deep relaxation and heightened awareness. Techniques range from focused attention meditation, in which practitioners focus on a single object or breath, to loving-kindness meditation, in which practitioners cultivate compassion for themselves and others. Meditation has been associated with better cognitive performance, emotional control, and a decrease in stress-related symptoms.

Mindfulness and meditation are frequently included in treatment strategies for ailments ranging from cardiovascular disease to chronic pain in integrative medicine. Mind-body programs that combine these techniques with traditional medical therapies are becoming increasingly common, indicating a growing awareness of the interdependence of mental and physical health. Scientific research into the neurological mechanisms underpinning the advantages of mindfulness and meditation continues, offering a growing evidence foundation for its inclusion in mainstream healthcare.

Yoga As A Therapeutic Method

Yoga, an ancient Indian practice, has evolved into a therapeutic method welcomed by integrative medicine because of its holistic approach to health. Yoga, in addition to its physical postures, or asanas, includes breath control (pranayama), meditation, and ethical ideals. Yoga can increase physical fitness, emotional well-being, and spiritual growth, according to integrative healthcare.

Numerous studies have shown that yoga can help with a variety of health issues, including cardiovascular disease, chronic pain, anxiety, and depression. The physical postures increase flexibility, strength, and balance, while the emphasis on breath awareness aids in stress reduction and relaxation. Yoga's meditative features can also improve mental clarity and emotional resilience.

The advent of specialized therapeutic yoga programs demonstrates yoga's acceptance into mainstream healthcare. These programs are frequently geared to treat specific health issues, such as back discomfort or cancer patients. The incorporation of yoga into standard medical settings demonstrates an understanding of its potential as a supplementary approach to existing therapies.

Integrative Pain Management Techniques

Chronic pain is a complicated and widespread health condition that frequently necessitates a diverse strategy for effective care. Integrative medicine provides pain treatment options that go beyond traditional pharmacological therapies. These treatments target not just the physical components of pain, but also the emotional and psychological issues that contribute to chronic pain experience.

Integrative pain care may comprise a combination of traditional medical treatments like pharmaceuticals and physical therapy as well as alternative therapies like acupuncture, massage, and mind-body approaches. Mindfulness-based therapies, cognitive-behavioral therapy, and relaxation methods are frequently used to assist people in managing pain-related stress and improving their overall quality of life.

The realization that pain is a subjective experience impacted by a variety of factors, including emotional well-being, lifestyle, and social support, is a critical component of integrative pain management. By treating underlying causes and improving self-care skills, this comprehensive approach strives to allow individuals to actively engage in their pain management.

Integrative pain treatment research is expanding, with studies investigating the efficacy of therapies such as yoga, acupuncture, and mindfulness for many types of pain disorders. The objective is to give individuals a variety of pain-management tools and techniques that are compatible with their preferences and beliefs.

Mental Health And Integrative Psychiatry

To address the complex character of mental health disorders, integrative psychiatry tries to combine standard psychiatric techniques with complementary and alternative therapies. Recognizing the interdependence of the mind and body, integrative psychiatry incorporates a variety of elements in the assessment and treatment of mental health illnesses, including biological, psychological, social, and spiritual components.

Integrative psychiatry combines evidence-based methods like psychotherapy and medication management with complementary therapies such as nutritional psychiatry, mindfulness-based interventions, and mind-body practices. Individualized care is prioritized, taking into account the unique biological and behavioral elements that contribute to each person's mental health difficulties.

A subspecialty of integrative psychiatry, nutritional psychiatry investigates the effects of food and nutrition on mental health. Certain food patterns and nutritional components, according to research, may impact mood, cognition, and general mental well-being. Integrative psychiatrists and nutritionists may collaborate to add dietary changes to the therapy approach.

Mind-body disciplines such as yoga, meditation, and relaxation methods are important in integrative psychiatry. These activities can aid in stress management, emotional control, and general resilience. Acupuncture, massage, and herbal supplements are examples of complementary therapies that integrative psychiatrists may investigate.

The integrated approach to mental health care represents a trend toward more comprehensive and patient-centered treatment strategies. Integrative psychiatry seeks to empower individuals in their mental health journeys and promote long-term well-being by taking into account the linked components of an individual's life.

Integrative Cancer Treatment

Integrative cancer care treats cancer in a complete and patient-centered manner, combining traditional medical approaches with complementary therapies to address the physical, emotional, and psychological components of the disease. This approach acknowledges that cancer affects the entire individual and that supportive care is critical throughout the cancer experience.

Acupuncture, massage, and mind-body practices are prominent complementary treatments used in cancer therapy to assist control of symptoms and enhance quality of life. These treatments may alleviate treatment-related adverse symptoms such as pain, exhaustion, anxiety, and nausea. To improve overall well-being, integrative cancer treatment stresses the need for dietary assistance, exercise, and psychological therapies.

Meditation and yoga, for example, play an important part in integrative cancer therapy by offering skills for stress reduction, improved sleep, and emotional well-being. These activities enable people to actively participate in their recovery process and deal with the emotional issues that come with a cancer diagnosis.

In integrated cancer care, nutritional therapies attempt to improve nutritional status during and after cancer therapy. Nutritionists may help people create tailored food programs that boost immune function, decrease inflammation, and enhance general health.

While integrative cancer care is gaining popularity, it is critical to combine these alternative techniques alongside evidence-based traditional treatments. Oncologists, integrative medicine practitioners, and other healthcare professionals work together to provide a coordinated and holistic approach to cancer care.

Finally, integrative medicine and mind-body healing provide a holistic and patient-centered approach to treatment. These techniques understand the interdependence of the body, mind, and spirit, from ancient wisdom in Ayurveda to current applications of mindfulness and meditation. Integrative medicine is not a replacement for traditional medical treatments, but rather a complementary and collaborative approach aimed at improving general well-being and empowering individuals on their health journey.

CHAPTER FOUR

Integrative Medicine's Spirituality And Healing

Integrative medicine acknowledges the interdependence of the mind, body, and spirit, recognizing that spiritual well-being is important for total health. Spirituality is a very personal and subjective experience that transcends religious connections, and it includes a sense of purpose, connection, and inner calm. Spirituality is interwoven into healthcare in the framework of integrative medicine to promote healing and improve the patient's general well-being.

Meditation, prayer, and mindfulness are all activities that connect spirituality with healing. These techniques are not only part of many ancient healing systems, but they have also acquired acceptance in modern healthcare due to their favorable influence on mental and physical health. Individuals who engage in regular spiritual activities have lower stress, better mental health, and more resilience in the face of sickness, according to research.

Integrative medicine practitioners collaborate with patients to investigate spiritual beliefs and incorporate them into treatment plans. To establish a more holistic and patient-centered care paradigm, this approach stresses the necessity of treating the spiritual dimension of health. Integrative medicine promotes an inclusive and culturally sensitive approach to healing by embracing and honoring varied spiritual beliefs.

Integrative medicine patients frequently experience a greater feeling of meaning and purpose in their lives. This spiritual component can bring consolation and support, especially during difficult times such as chronic disease or surgical recovery. Integrative medicine seeks to establish a therapeutic environment that nurtures not just the physical body but also the spirit, acknowledging that a balanced and harmonious link between mind, body, and spirit is necessary for total well-being.

Pediatric Integrative Care

Integrative pediatric care is a comprehensive approach to children's health that incorporates mainstream medicine as well as complementary and alternative therapies.

Recognizing children's special requirements, integrative pediatric treatment focuses on general well-being, disease prevention, and supporting the body's natural healing processes. This method is very useful in dealing with chronic diseases, developmental problems, and behavioral challenges in young patients.

The emphasis on preventative techniques, such as diet, physical exercise, and stress management, is an important part of integrative pediatric treatment. Integrative pediatric care aims to promote optimal growth and development by addressing lifestyle variables at a young age, building the groundwork for a healthy future.

Collaboration between healthcare practitioners, parents, and other caregivers is required to provide a supportive environment for children's well-being.

Acupuncture, chiropractic therapy, and herbal medicine may be incorporated into the treatment plan, offering additional options to address a variety of pediatric health conditions. Integrative pediatric care understands that children's responses to traditional treatments may vary, and adding complementary therapies allows for a more tailored and patient-centered approach.

Furthermore, integrated pediatric care emphasizes the need to integrate families in decision-making. Parents and caregivers are seen as crucial participants in their child's healthcare journey, and their participation is appreciated in developing a thorough and personalized care plan. This collaborative approach generates a sense of empowerment and involvement, which improves the treatment's overall success.

Preventive Medicine And Lifestyle Medicine

Lifestyle medicine is a subspecialty of integrative medicine that focuses on resolving the underlying causes of chronic illnesses via long-term lifestyle changes. Many health issues, such as heart disease, diabetes, and obesity, are connected to lifestyle variables such as nutrition, physical exercise, sleep, and stress. Lifestyle medicine tries to prevent and even reverse chronic illnesses by making focused adjustments in these areas, improving long-term health and well-being.

Preventive healthcare is a key component of lifestyle medicine, emphasizing the necessity of taking proactive steps to preserve good health and avoid sickness. This approach differs from standard healthcare practices, which frequently focus on treating symptoms as they emerge. Instead, lifestyle medicine encourages people to develop healthy behaviors and make educated decisions that benefit their entire health.

Personalized therapies are critical in lifestyle medicine. Individuals engage with healthcare specialists to examine their specific lifestyle characteristics and build personalized plans for change. Nutritional advice, exercise regimens, stress management strategies, and sleep hygiene may all be included.

The objective is to inspire people to take an active part in their health and implement long-term lifestyle changes that help avoid disease.

Lifestyle medicine's incorporation into mainstream healthcare signifies a paradigm shift toward a more holistic and patient-centered approach. It acknowledges the interdependence of many lifestyle variables and their influence on health outcomes. Lifestyle medicine strives to decrease dependency on pharmaceuticals and medical treatments by treating the fundamental causes of chronic illnesses and advocating a more natural and sustainable approach to health.

Integrative Treatments For Chronic Diseases

Integrative medicine provides a holistic and patient-centered approach to chronic illness management. Integrative treatments, rather than focusing primarily on symptom management, seek to discover and treat the underlying causes of chronic diseases, promoting long-term healing and well-being. This method is very useful in the treatment of diabetes, cardiovascular disease, and autoimmune illnesses.

The emphasis on tailored treatment regimens is a significant feature of integrative treatments for chronic illnesses. Healthcare practitioners work with individuals to learn about their own health history, lifestyle, and preferences. This tailored approach enables focused therapies that address the individual elements that contribute to chronic illness, resulting in more effective and long-term outcomes.

Acupuncture, massage, and mind-body practices may be included in the treatment plan to improve general well-being and reduce symptoms.

These therapies go beyond typical medical interventions by recognizing the interdependence of physical, mental, and emotional health. Integrative medicine strives to enhance the quality of life for those living with chronic conditions by addressing the complete person.

Integrative methods also highlight the significance of lifestyle changes in the management of chronic illnesses. A complete treatment strategy includes nutrition, exercise, stress management, and sleep hygiene. Integrative medicine strives to increase total health and resilience in the face of chronic disease by empowering patients to make positive changes in these areas.

CHAPTER FIVE

Integrative Stress Reduction Therapies

Stress is a common occurrence in modern life, and its negative influence on health is widely established. Integrative medicine provides several therapies to address and lessen the consequences of stress, acknowledging the connectivity of the mind and body in the stress response. These integrative therapies seek to improve not just stress symptoms but also general well-being and resilience.

Mind-body practices such as meditation, mindfulness, and yoga play an important part in integrative stress reduction therapy. These techniques have been demonstrated to modify the body's stress response, resulting in lower stress hormone levels and better overall mental and physical health. Integrative medicine acknowledges the necessity of implementing these practices into everyday life to increase resilience and cope with stress.

Massage therapy, acupuncture, and aromatherapy are examples of complementary treatments that can be used in conjunction with stress reduction strategies. These techniques not only give physical relaxation but also help with mental well-being. Integrative medicine sees stress reduction as a multifaceted undertaking that addresses both the physical and emotional elements of stress to foster a balanced and resilient response to life's challenges.

Counseling and psychotherapy are also important components of integrative stress management treatments. These techniques assist individuals in identifying the underlying causes of stress, developing coping skills, and cultivating a positive mentality.

Integrative medicine strives to produce long-term improvements that enhance general mental and emotional well-being by addressing the underlying psychological problems that contribute to stress.

The Mind-Body Connection In Science

A basic premise underpinning integrative medicine is the science of the mind-body link. This notion acknowledges that the mind and body are inextricably linked, with one having a significant influence on the other. Scientific study has shed light on how mental and emotional emotions may affect physical health by providing insights into the complicated interactions between the brain, nervous system, and numerous physiological systems.

The function of stress in contributing to a wide range of health issues is an important part of the mind-body link. Chronic stress has been related to heart disease, immune system malfunction, and inflammatory diseases. Understanding the physiological processes by which stress affects the body enables the creation of specific therapies to ameliorate these effects, highlighting the relevance of stress reduction in integrative medicine.

Another area of study in the science of the mind-body relationship is neuroplasticity, or the brain's ability to restructure and adapt. This phenomenon underpins the possibility of good changes in mental and emotional states that may be achieved via techniques like meditation and mindfulness. According to research, these mind-body practices can cause structural changes in the brain, therefore improving emotional control, cognitive performance, and general well-being.

The mind-body link is also important in the placebo effect, which occurs when belief and anticipation impact the body's reaction to therapy. Integrative medicine understands the importance of utilizing the mind's healing capacity and integrates treatments that positively leverage the placebo effect.

Mind-body therapy, supportive communication, and the creation of healing settings are examples of how to improve the overall efficacy of treatments.

Finally, integrated medicine recognizes the mind, body, and spirit's inherent interdependence. Integrative medicine's primary ideas include a holistic and patient-centered approach to healthcare, from spirituality and healing to pediatric care, lifestyle medicine, and approaches to chronic illnesses and stress reduction. Integrative medicine strives to promote healing, prevent illness, and improve general well-being by combining complementary treatments, tailored treatment regimens, and an emphasis on the mind-body link.

Integrative Medicine Research And Evidence

Integrative medicine has grown in popularity in recent years as a comprehensive approach that blends traditional medicine with complementary and alternative therapies. One important part of its credibility and efficacy is study and proof. Traditional medicine frequently uses randomized controlled trials (RCTs) to determine therapy effectiveness. However, because of its diverse and customized nature, integrative medicine confronts issues in integrating into this standard research approach.

Integrative medicine research frequently uses a combination of qualitative and quantitative methodologies. Observational studies, case studies, and cohort studies are critical for understanding the real-world complexity of integrative techniques. For example, mindfulness-based therapies for chronic pain can be evaluated using both clinical outcomes and patient-reported experiences, allowing for a more complete knowledge of therapy effects.

The variety of therapies and patient demographics is one issue in integrative medicine research. Integrative medicine includes herbal medicine, acupuncture, mind-body practices, and nutritional therapy. It is critical to tailor research approaches to certain modalities and situations. Certain therapies are progressively gaining support, such as the beneficial benefits of acupuncture on pain and nausea or mindfulness-based stress reduction in mental health.

Advances in neuroimaging and molecular biology have also added to the evidence foundation for integrated medicine. Functional magnetic resonance imaging (fMRI) and genomics research shed light on the physiological underpinnings behind mind-body treatments. These technologies add to the expanding body of research that supports the incorporation of alternative medicines into standard healthcare.

Despite advancements, standardizing research procedures and guaranteeing methodological rigor remain obstacles.

The field must develop unambiguous outcome measurements, address placebo effects, and employ rigorous study methods. Collaboration between conventional medical researchers and practitioners of complementary therapies is also critical for improving integrated medicine research.

Integrating Complementary And Alternative Medicine Into Conventional Medicine

Integrative medicine tries to bridge the gap between traditional and supplementary medical treatments. The combination of these two techniques has the potential to improve patient care by delivering a more thorough and tailored treatment plan.

Communication and teamwork among healthcare professionals is an important part of integration. An open discussion between conventional physicians and complementary therapy practitioners is critical for assessing the patient's overall health and developing a coherent treatment approach. This multidisciplinary approach guarantees that patients get the best of both worlds, receiving evidence-based treatment as well as alternative therapies suited to their specific requirements.

Another important aspect of effective integration is education. Healthcare providers must be aware of the data supporting complementary medicines as well as their possible interactions with conventional treatments. To minimize harmful effects or conflicts, complementary medicine practitioners should be informed of the patient's medical history as well as any continuing conventional therapy.

In certain circumstances, integrated medicine involves sequential therapy, which entails introducing complementary therapies following conventional treatments to alleviate remaining symptoms or enhance general well-being. Cancer patients, for example, who are receiving chemotherapy, may benefit from acupuncture to decrease treatment-related adverse effects.

Patient involvement is critical in the integration of alternative treatments. Giving patients information about different treatment alternatives helps them to actively participate in decision-making. Sharing decision-making between healthcare practitioners and patients promotes a more patient-centered approach, which leads to better treatment adherence and results.

However, there are obstacles to incorporating complementary medicines, such as varied levels of evidence, cultural differences, and possible mistrust among healthcare practitioners. To assist the integration process and assure patient safety, standardized standards and practices are required. Furthermore, continued research and teaching initiatives are required to provide a solid evidence foundation and improve awareness of how various treatments might supplement traditional therapy.

CHAPTER SIX

Integrative Medicine Provides Patient-Centered Care

The notion of patient-centered treatment, which prioritizes the individual's preferences, values, and objectives in the decision-making process, is central to integrative medicine. This approach respects the individuality of each patient and seeks to address not only the symptoms but also the individual's total well-being.

The emphasis in patient-centered treatment within integrative medicine is on developing a therapeutic partnership between the healthcare professional and the patient. This collaboration entails open communication, shared decision-making, and a team-based approach to treatment planning. Patients are encouraged to communicate their preferences, concerns, and expectations, resulting in a more individualized and holistic healthcare experience.

Longer consultation sessions are common in integrative medicine, allowing healthcare experts to dig into patients' lives, stresses, and personal views about health and sickness. This thorough understanding allows for the creation of personalized treatment regimens that incorporate both traditional medical procedures and alternative therapies.

The encouragement of self-care and patient empowerment is another important part of patient-centered treatment in integrative medicine. Patients are instructed on lifestyle changes, stress management strategies, and complementary therapies that are appropriate for their needs. This method promotes autonomy and encourages individuals to actively engage in their rehabilitation.

Despite its numerous advantages, patient-centered treatment in integrative medicine has several problems, including time restrictions, funding concerns, and the requirement for interdisciplinary teamwork.

Healthcare systems must evolve to accommodate extended consultation hours and understand the need for full patient evaluations. Furthermore, continuing education for healthcare personnel is essential for improving their communication, cultural competency, and integrative medicine modalities.

Integrative Healthcare's Difficulties And Debates

While integrative healthcare has the potential to provide a more holistic and tailored approach to treatment, it is not without its obstacles and debates. The lack of standards in the sector is a big obstacle. The wide variety of complementary therapies, variable degrees of evidence, and unique treatment regimens make developing uniform standards challenging.

Disagreements can develop as a result of the incorporation of therapies with weak scientific evidence into mainstream healthcare. certain critics contend that certain complementary treatments lack strong evidence and may potentially endanger patients. Patient safety is critical, and integrative medicine must strike a delicate balance between innovation and evidence-based practice.

Additional obstacles are posed by financial considerations and reimbursement issues. Integrative healthcare frequently entails extended consultation hours, different therapy modalities, and tailored treatment plans, which may or may not be compatible with the standard fee-for-service paradigm. This calls into question the economic viability of integrative techniques and their inclusion into conventional healthcare systems.

Another barrier is skepticism among healthcare practitioners and the general public. Many medical professionals may be unfamiliar with or suspicious of complementary therapies, resulting in a lack of faith in integrative medicine.

Public education and awareness initiatives are critical for dispelling myths and instilling trust in the safety and efficacy of integrative medicine.

Interdisciplinary collaboration is essential for successful integrative healthcare, yet it can be difficult to achieve smooth communication and cooperation between traditional medical specialists and alternative practitioners. Bridging the educational and communication styles divide is critical for developing a coherent and patient-centered strategy.

Addressing these issues would need continual study, education, and policy creation. Standardizing integrative medicine education for healthcare practitioners, providing clear rules for the integration of complementary medicines, and addressing reimbursement models are essential steps toward overcoming difficulties and supporting integrative healthcare growth.

Integrative Medicine's Future Trends

Integrative medicine's environment is always changing, with various developing themes determining its future. These developments show a rising appreciation for the value of holistic and patient-centered approaches to healthcare.

1. Advances in genetics, molecular biology, and data analytics are paving the path for customized and precision integrative care. Individualizing therapies based on genetic composition, lifestyle, and environmental variables will become more widespread, improving therapeutic outcomes.

2. Integration of Technology: The integration of technology, such as mobile health applications, wearables, and telehealth platforms, will be critical in the future of integrative medicine.

These technologies will improve patient participation, allow for real-time monitoring, and allow for remote consultations with integrative healthcare practitioners.

3. Expansion of Mind-Body Medicine: The mind-body link will continue to gain traction in integrative medicine. As evidence for the effectiveness of mindfulness-based therapies, meditation, and yoga

accumulates, they will become more generally acknowledged. Integrative treatments for mental health and stress-related diseases will be on the cutting edge of innovation.

4. Collaboration and Interdisciplinary Training: Future healthcare professionals will get greater interdisciplinary training, increasing collaboration between conventional and alternative practitioners. This will lead to improved communication, comprehension, and integration of various treatment modalities into patient care.

5. Health System Integration: Integrative medicine will become more prevalent in mainstream healthcare systems. To deliver more complete and patient-centered treatment within traditional medical settings, collaborative models that integrate conventional and alternative therapies will be devised.

6. Research Advances: Ongoing research will fill gaps in the evidence foundation of integrative

medicine. Extensive research into the mechanisms of action, safety, and efficacy of complementary medicines will help to provide a more solid scientific foundation for integrative methods.

7. Patient Empowerment and Education: In integrated medicine, there will be a stronger emphasis on patient empowerment and education. Patients will take a more active part in their healthcare decisions, selecting conventional and alternative therapies based on their interests and beliefs.

8. Global Integration of Traditional Medicine: Traditional healing techniques from diverse cultures throughout the world will be progressively included in integrative medicine. This worldwide integration will increase the variety of therapeutic alternatives accessible and contribute to a more inclusive approach to healthcare.

While these trends bode well for the future of integrative medicine, resolving obstacles and disputes, stimulating research, and fostering education will be critical for the holistic approach to healing's sustained expansion and acceptance. Integrative medicine's promise to enhance patient outcomes and general well-being will be realized on a larger scale when it becomes more thoroughly embedded in healthcare systems.

Conclusion

Integrative medicine and mind-body therapy, in conclusion, reflect a comprehensive approach to healthcare that recognizes the interdependence of the mind, body, and spirit.

This paradigm shift in medical thought emphasizes that achieving optimal health needs a thorough awareness of the individual's mental, emotional, and spiritual well-being, rather than focusing simply on physical symptoms.

Integrative medicine encompasses a wide range of therapies, such as standard Western medicine, complementary and alternative practices, and mind-body approaches including meditation, yoga, and mindfulness. The combination of these treatments promotes a patient-centered model that allows people to actively engage in their healing.

According to research in this discipline, incorporating mind-body techniques into traditional medical care can improve overall health outcomes, reduce stress, and improve chronic disease management.

The emphasis on prevention, wellness, and the importance of the mind in healing reflects a shift from traditional medicine's reactive character, creating a proactive and collaborative approach to treatment.

As the medical world continues to investigate and adopt integrative treatments, it is clear that treating the complete person, rather than simply the disease, is critical for reaching real well-being.

Integrative medicine and mind-body healing hold great potential for the future of healthcare by providing a more complete and compassionate approach to treatment that recognizes the complexities of the human experience.

THE END